THE PICTURE BOOK OF

BIBLE VERSES

I0419544

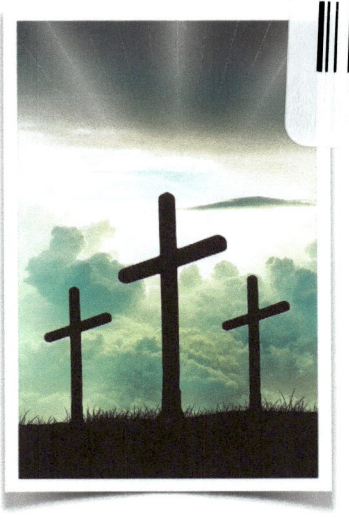

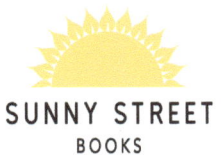

SUNNY STREET
BOOKS

Your word is a lamp

to my feet and a

light to my path.

Psalms 119:105

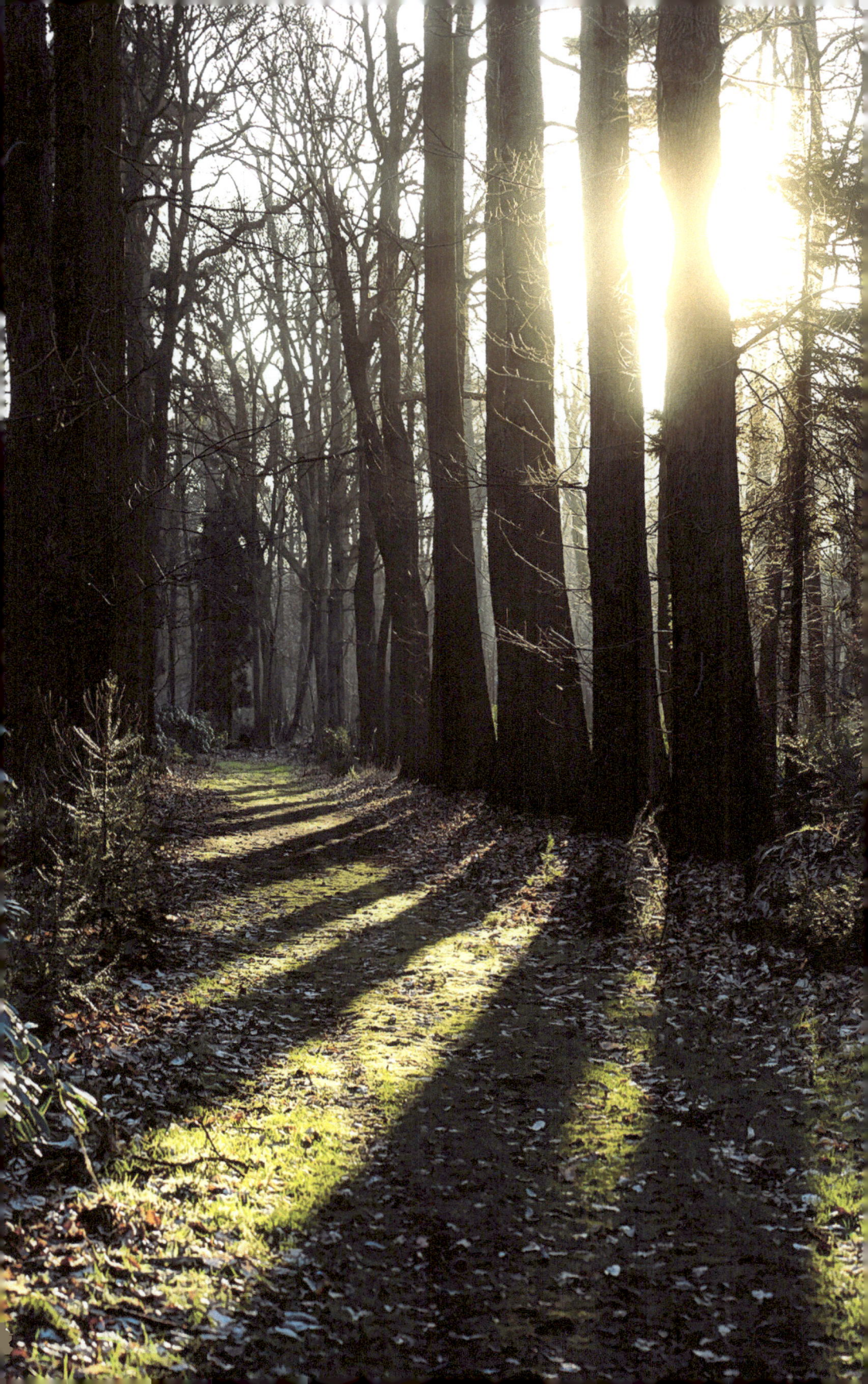

God is with you

wherever you go.

Joshua 1:9

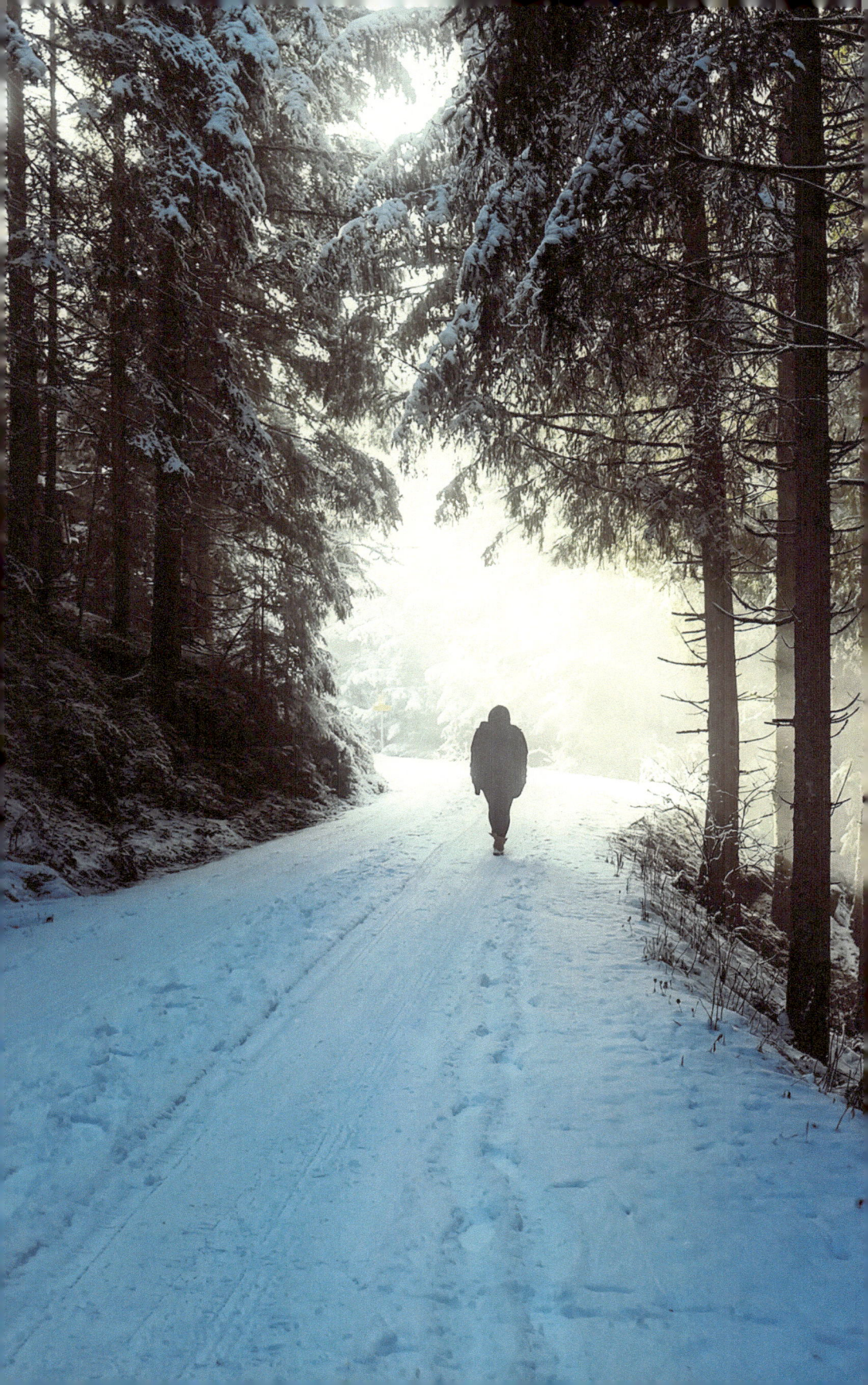

We love because

He first loved us.

John 4:19

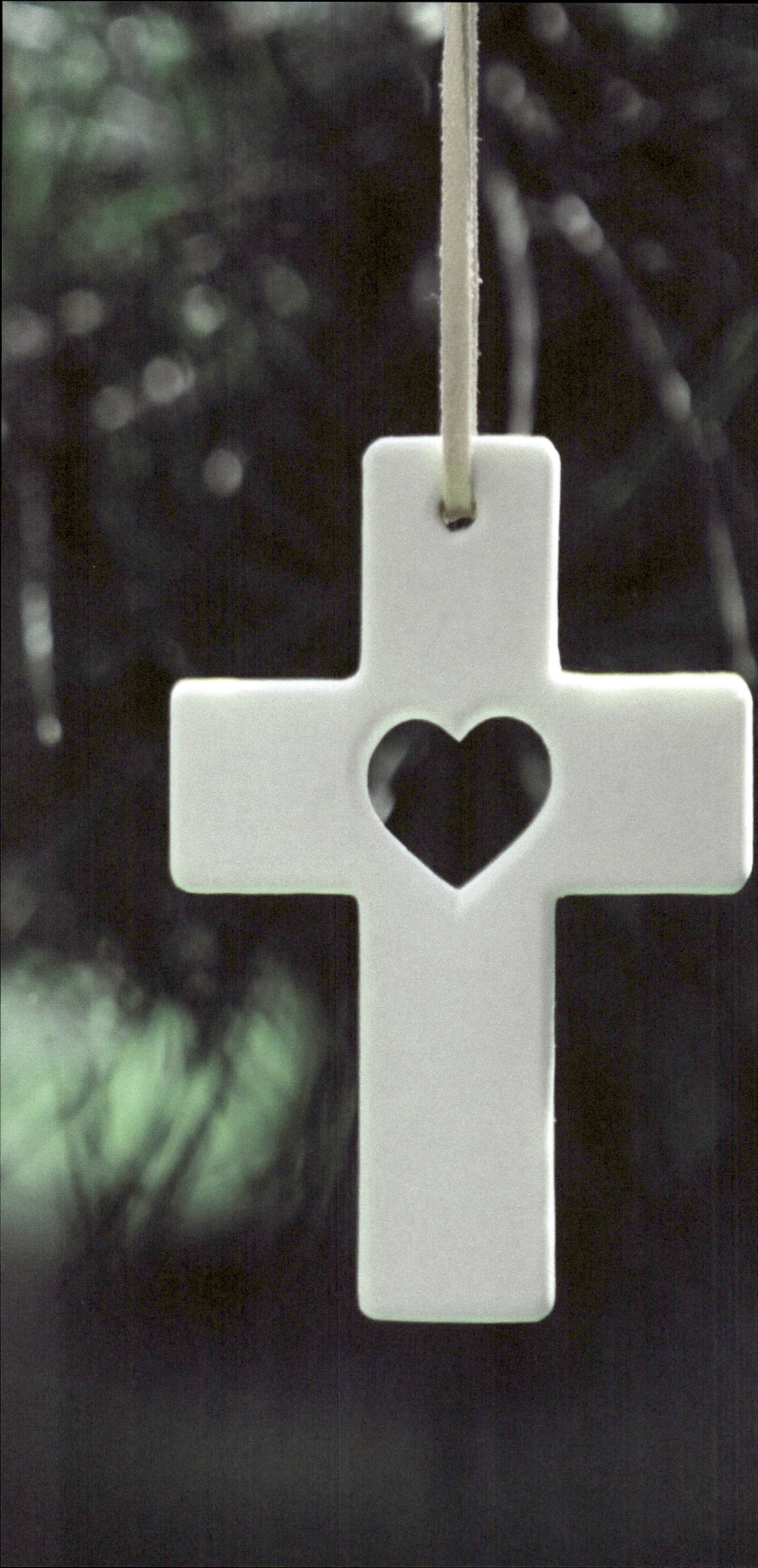

When you pass

through the waters,

I will be with you.

Isaiah 43:2

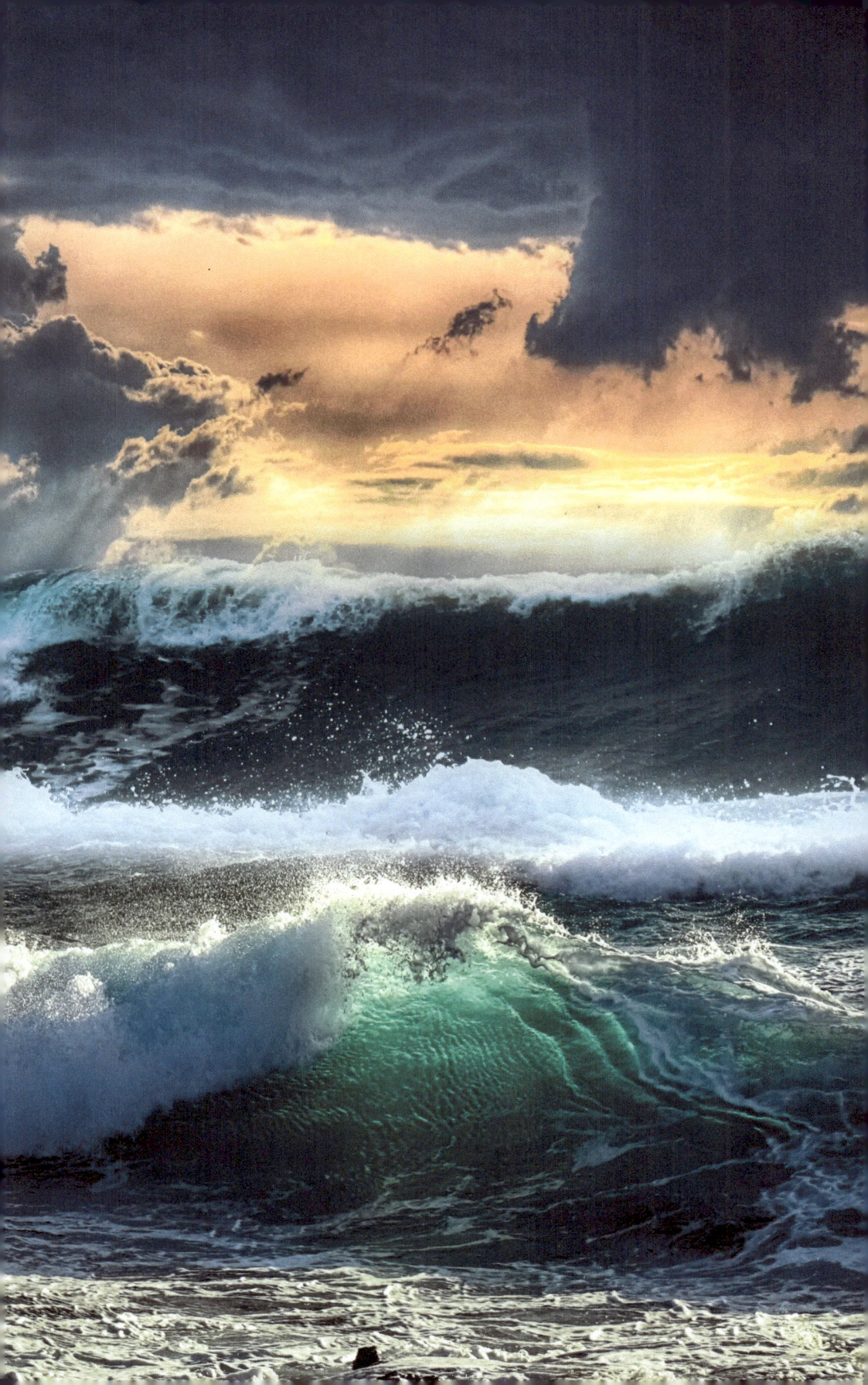

Set your mind on
things above, not on
earthly things.

Colossians 3:2

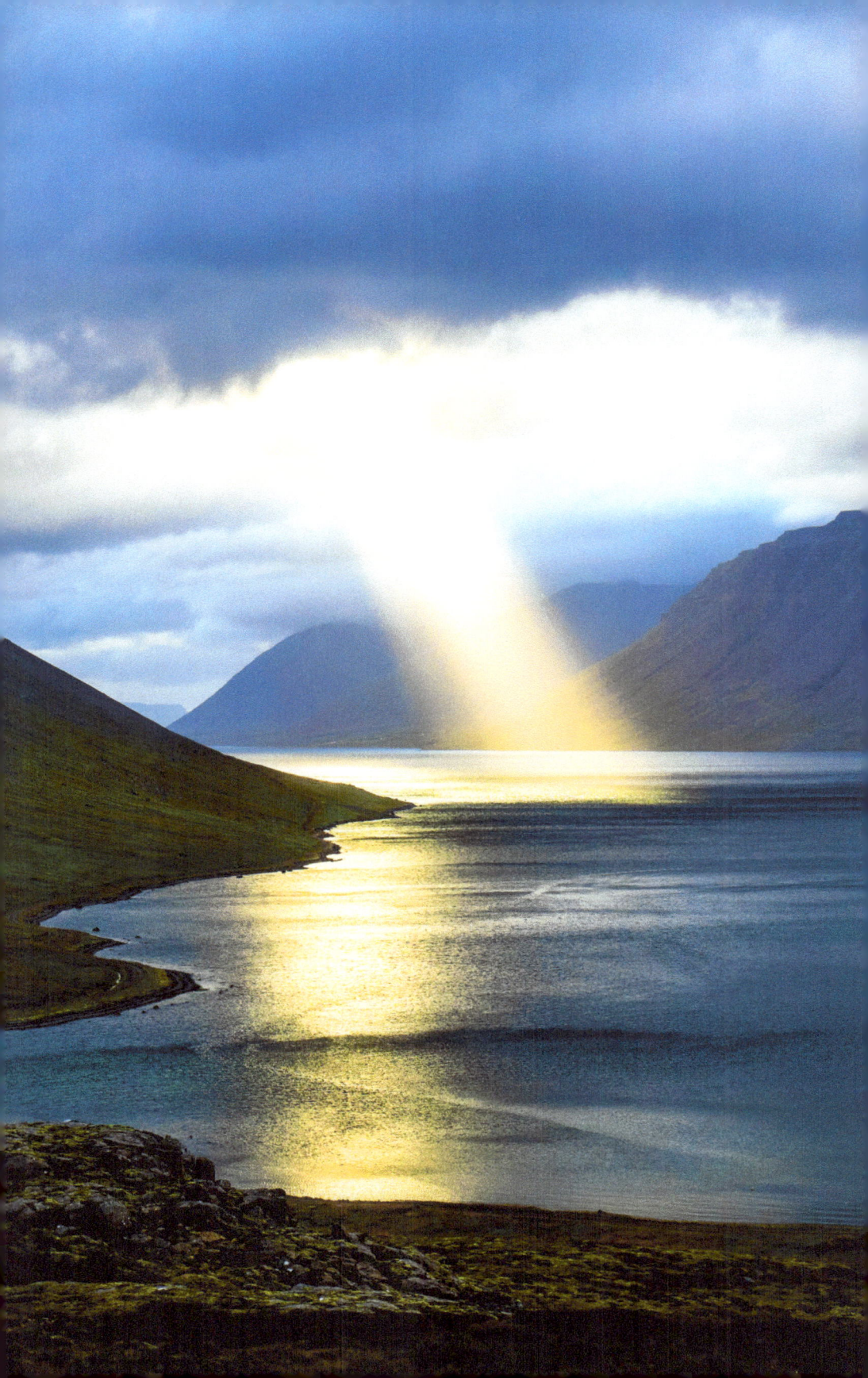

The Lord is my

light and my

salvation.

Psalms 27:1

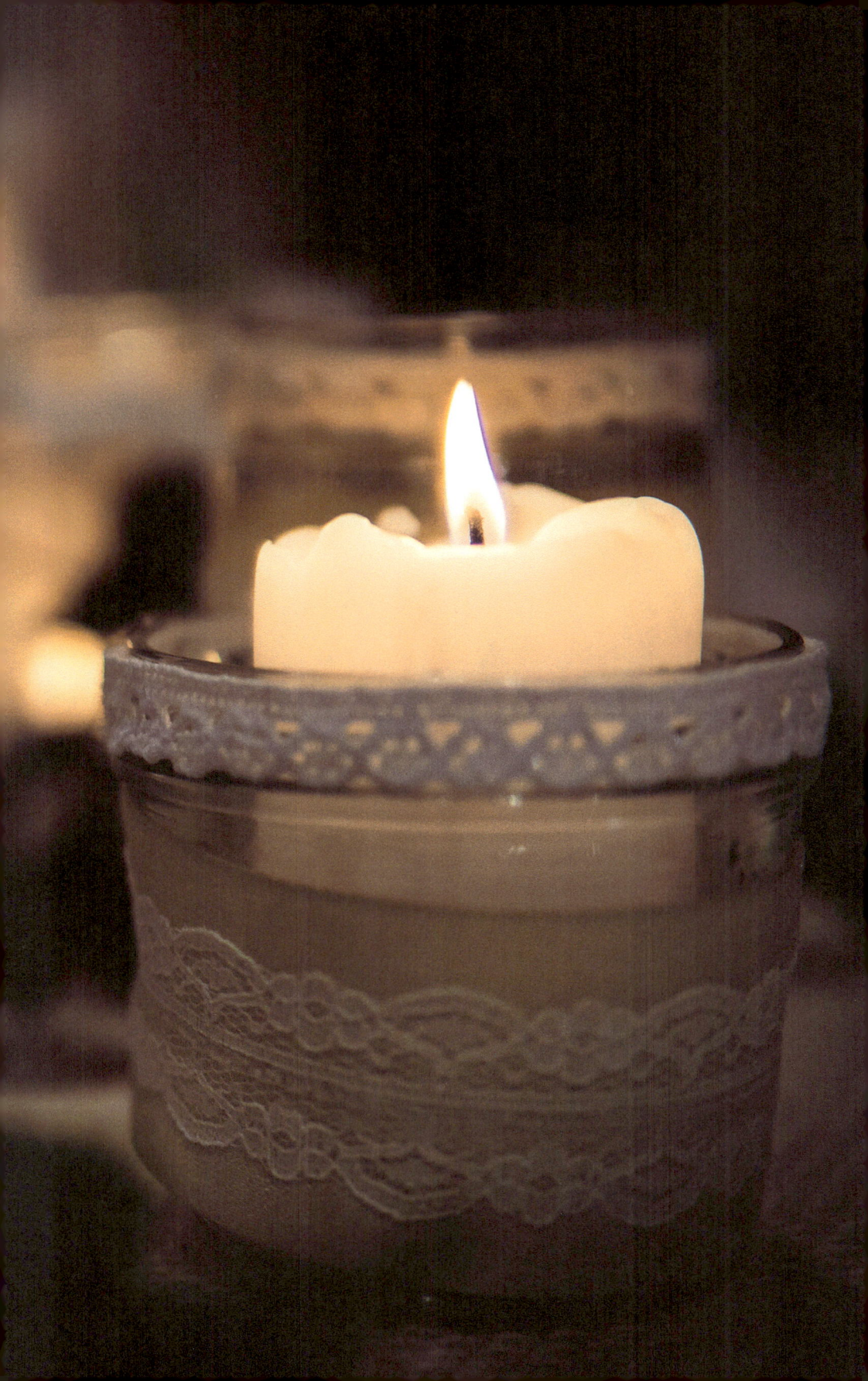

When I am afraid,

I put my trust

in God.

Psalms 56:3

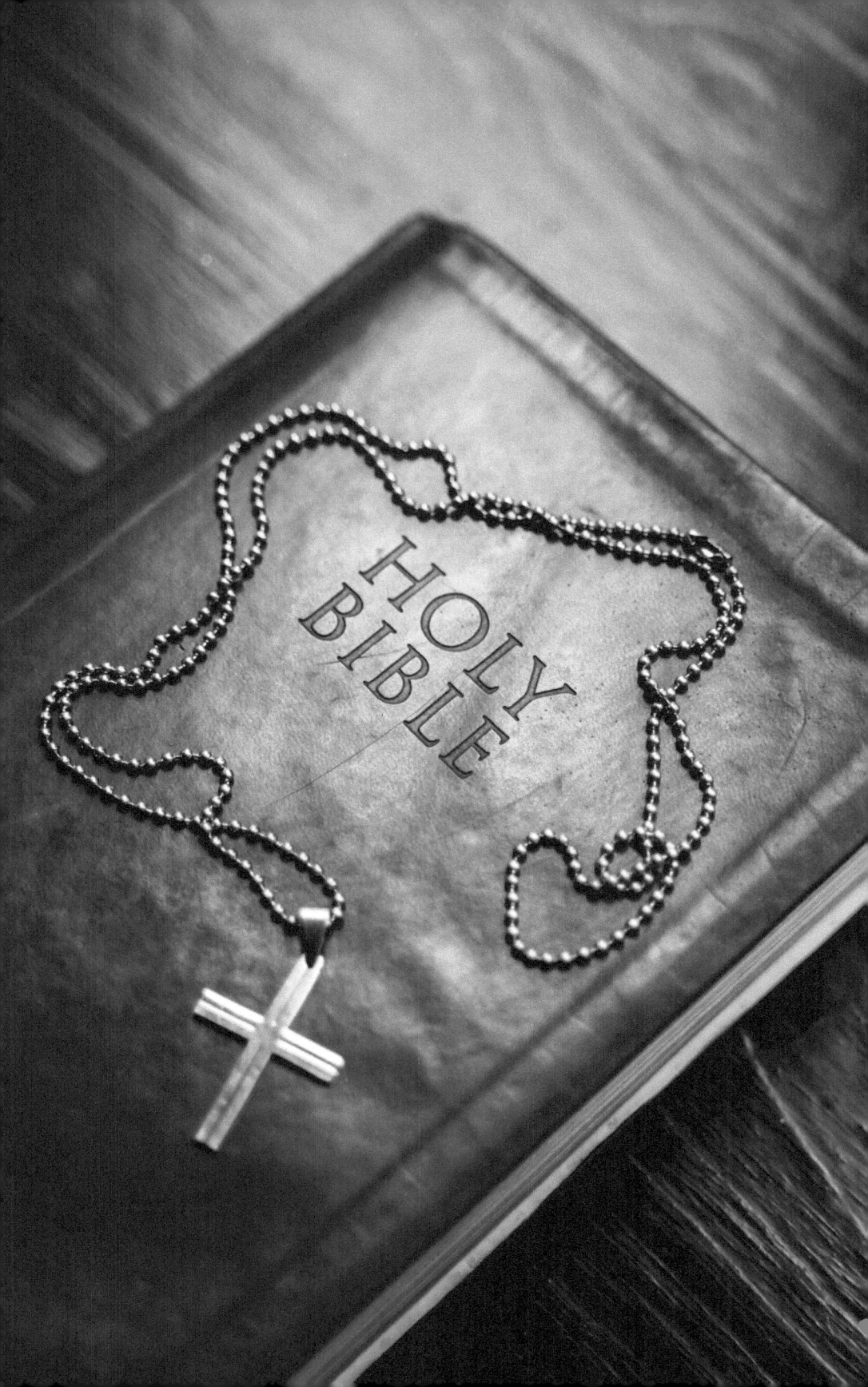

Rejoice in the
Lord always.

Philippians 4:4

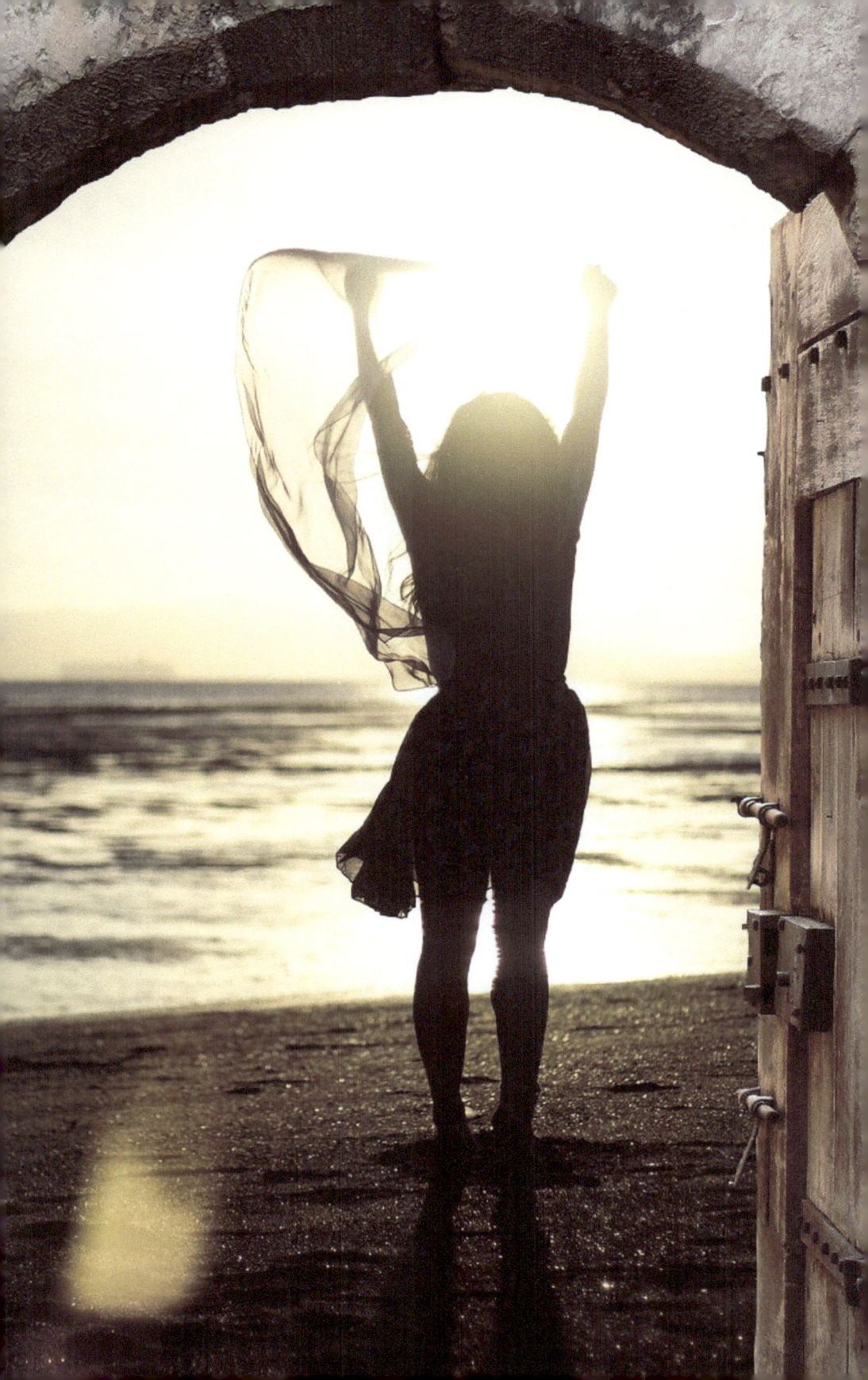

May the God of

hope fill you with

love and peace.

Romans 15:13

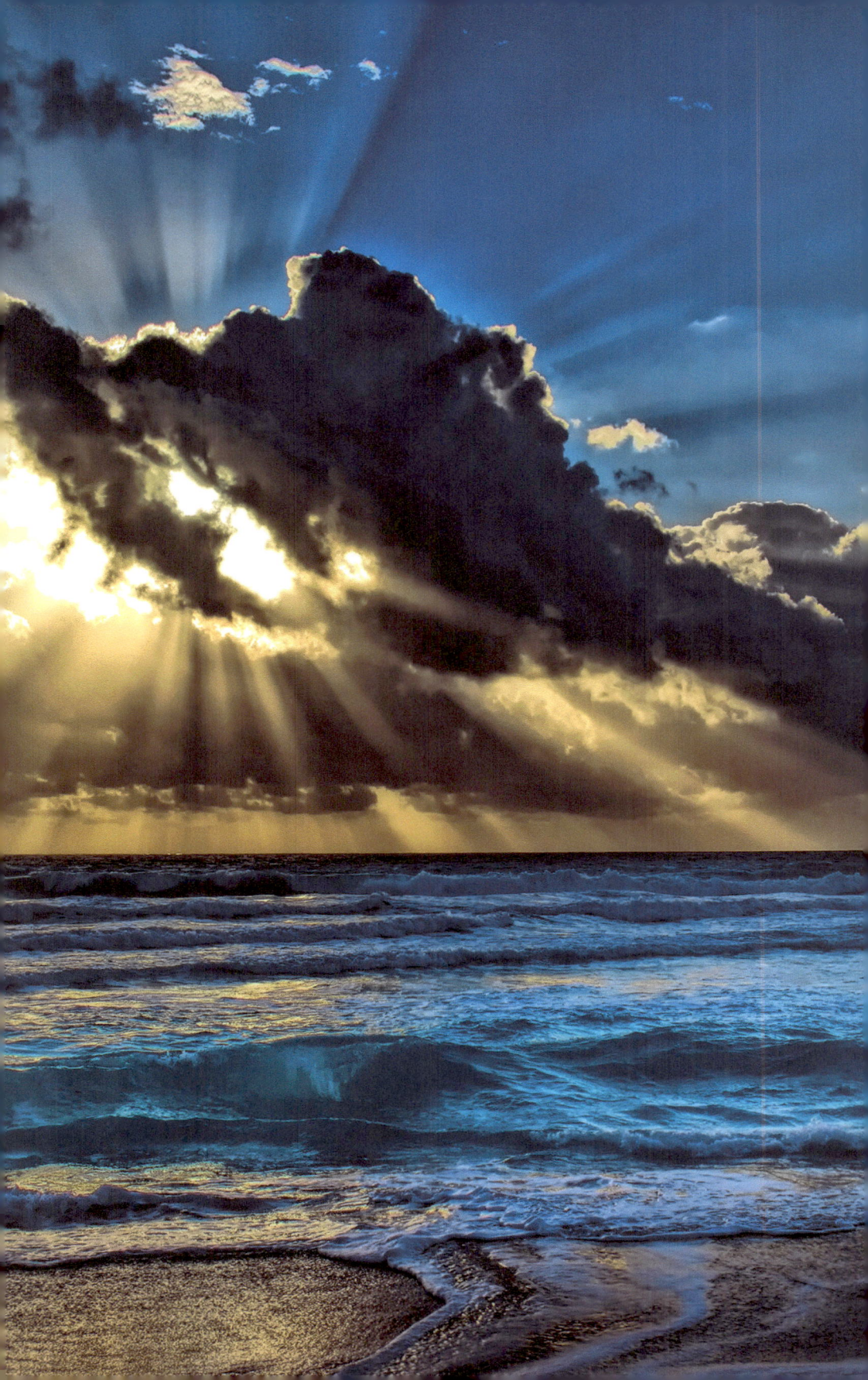

The Lord is my
shepherd, I shall
not want.

Psalms 27:1

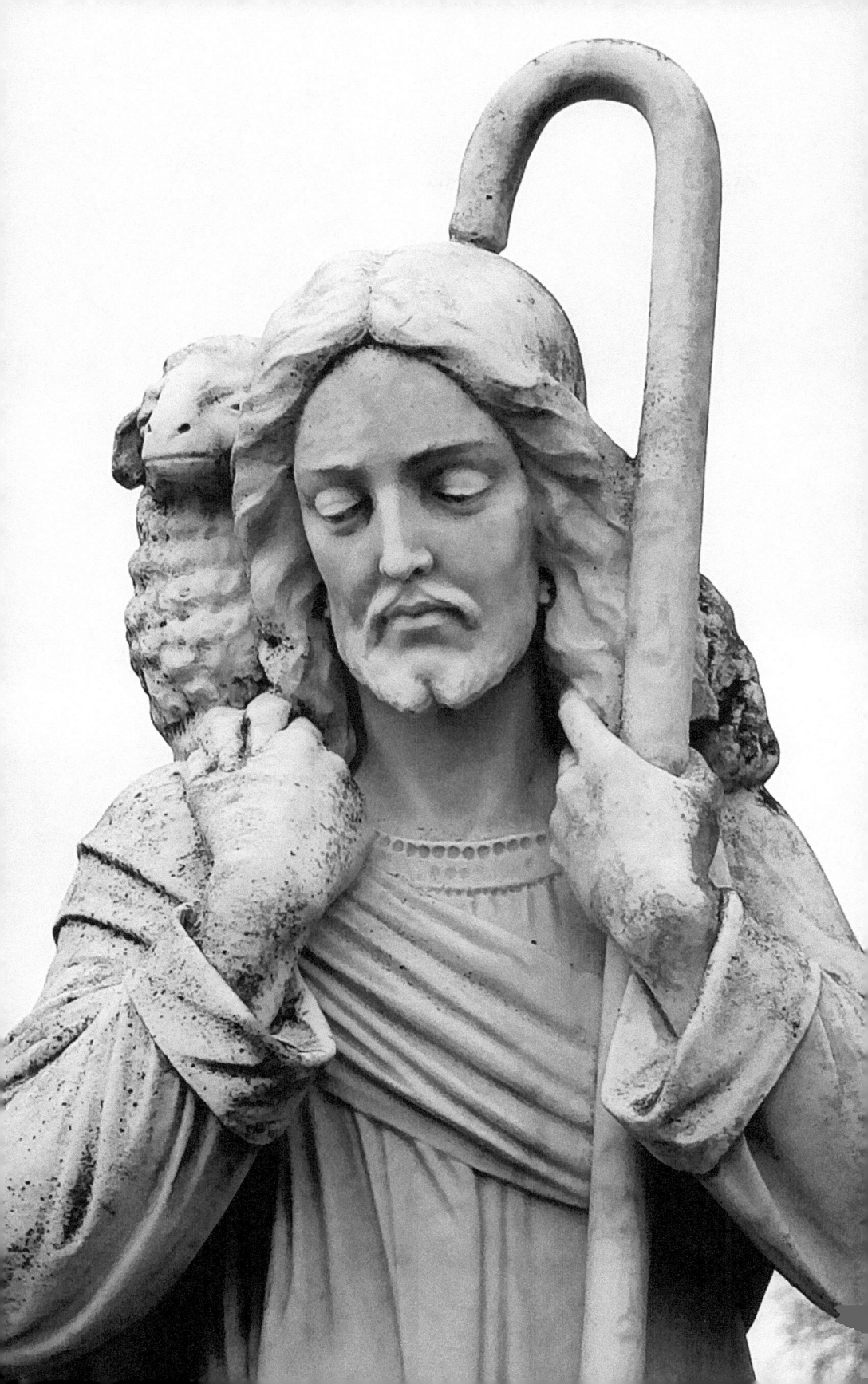

A friend loves

at all times.

*P*roverbs 17:17

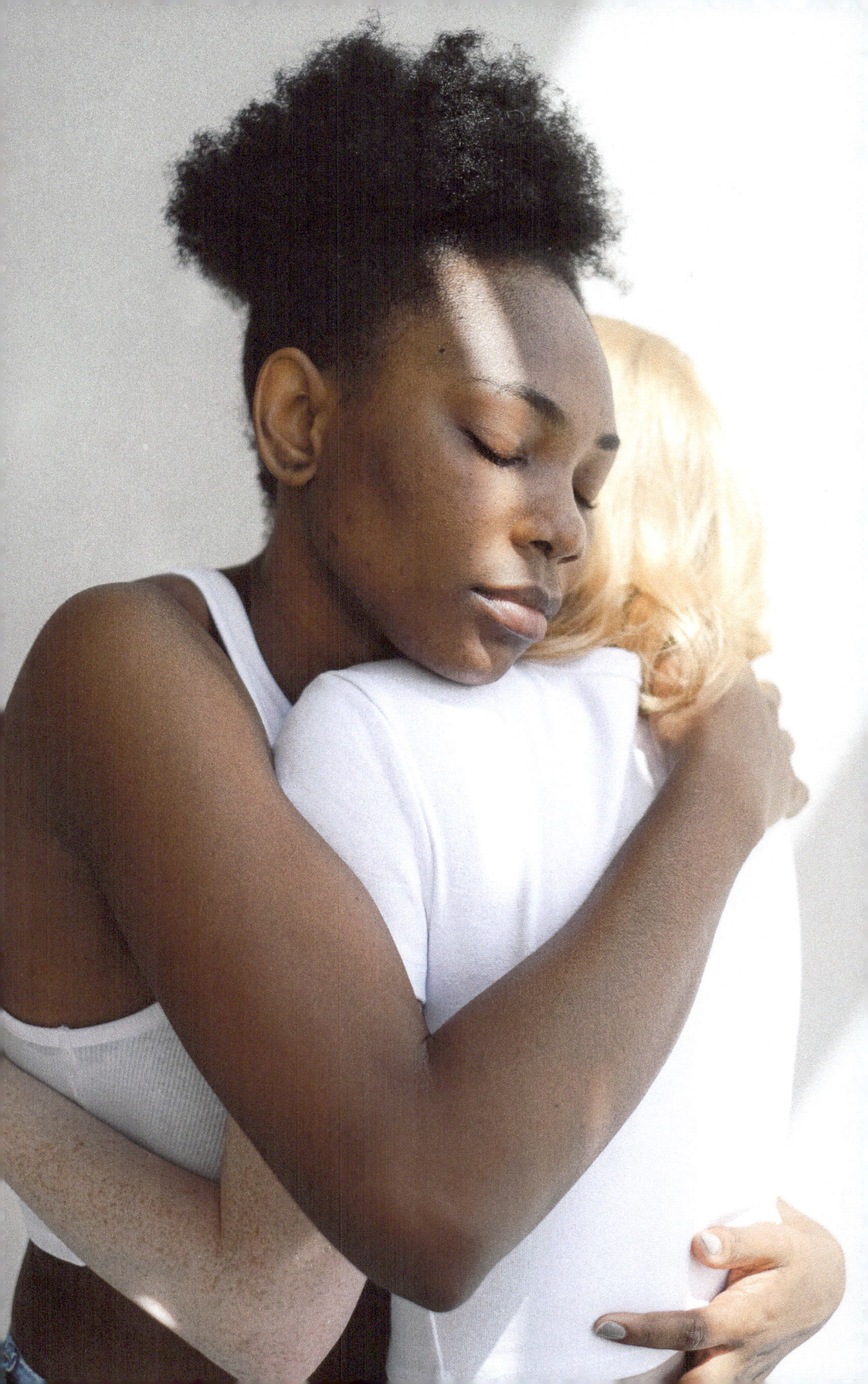

Believe in the

Lord Jesus and

you will be saved.

Acts 16:31

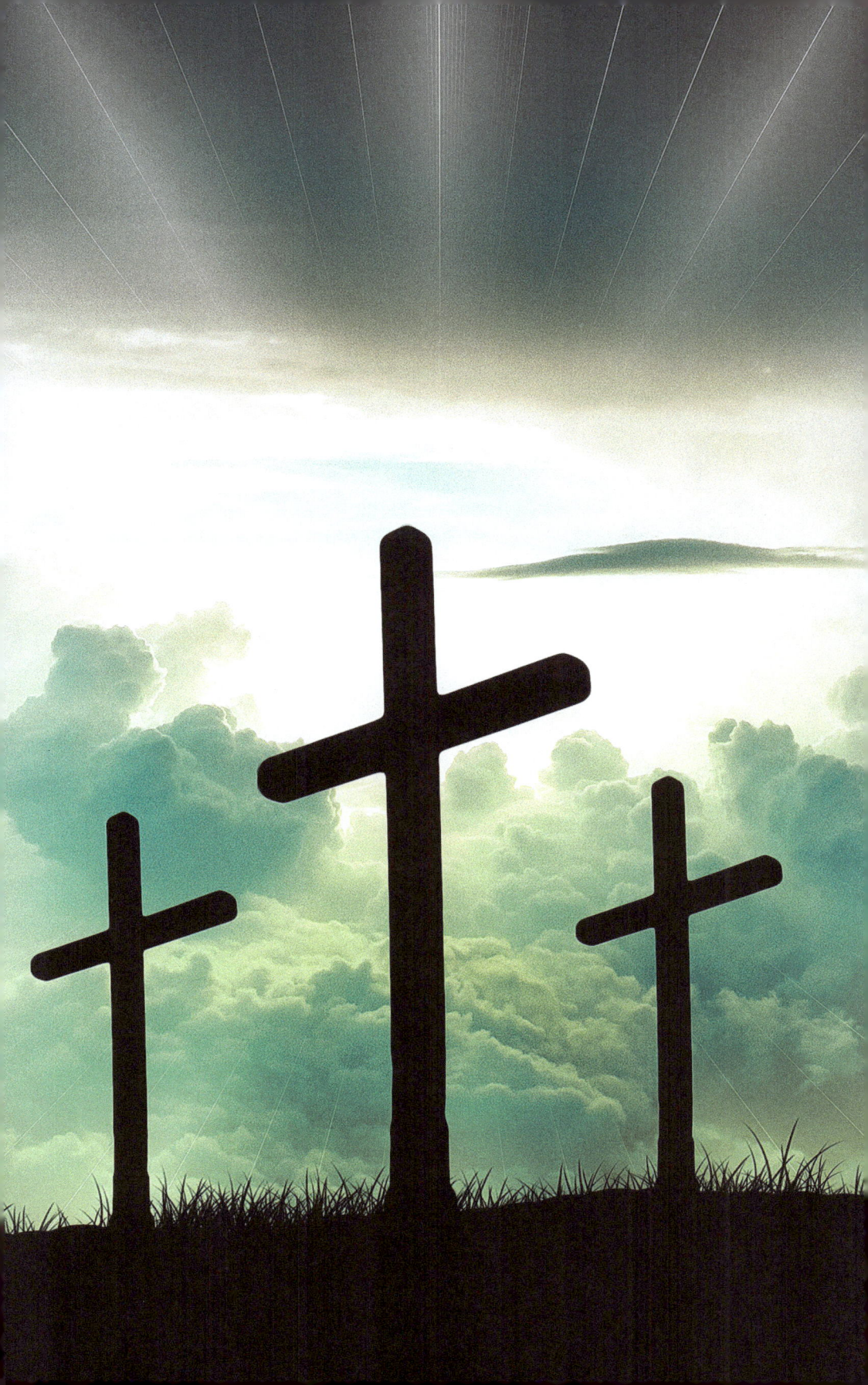

Trust in the Lord

with all your heart.

Proverbs 3:5

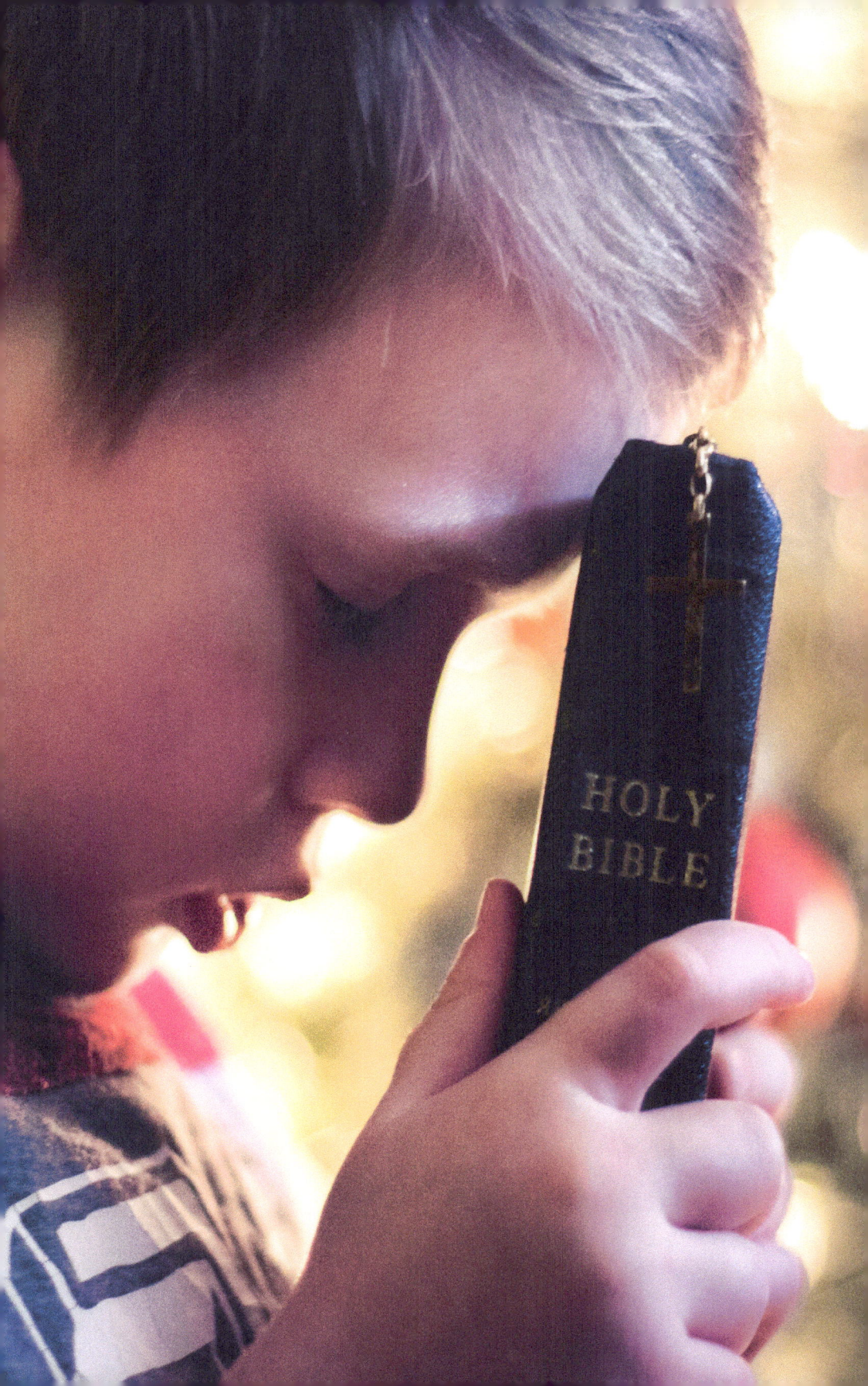

The Lord is my rock

and my fortress.

Psalm 18:2

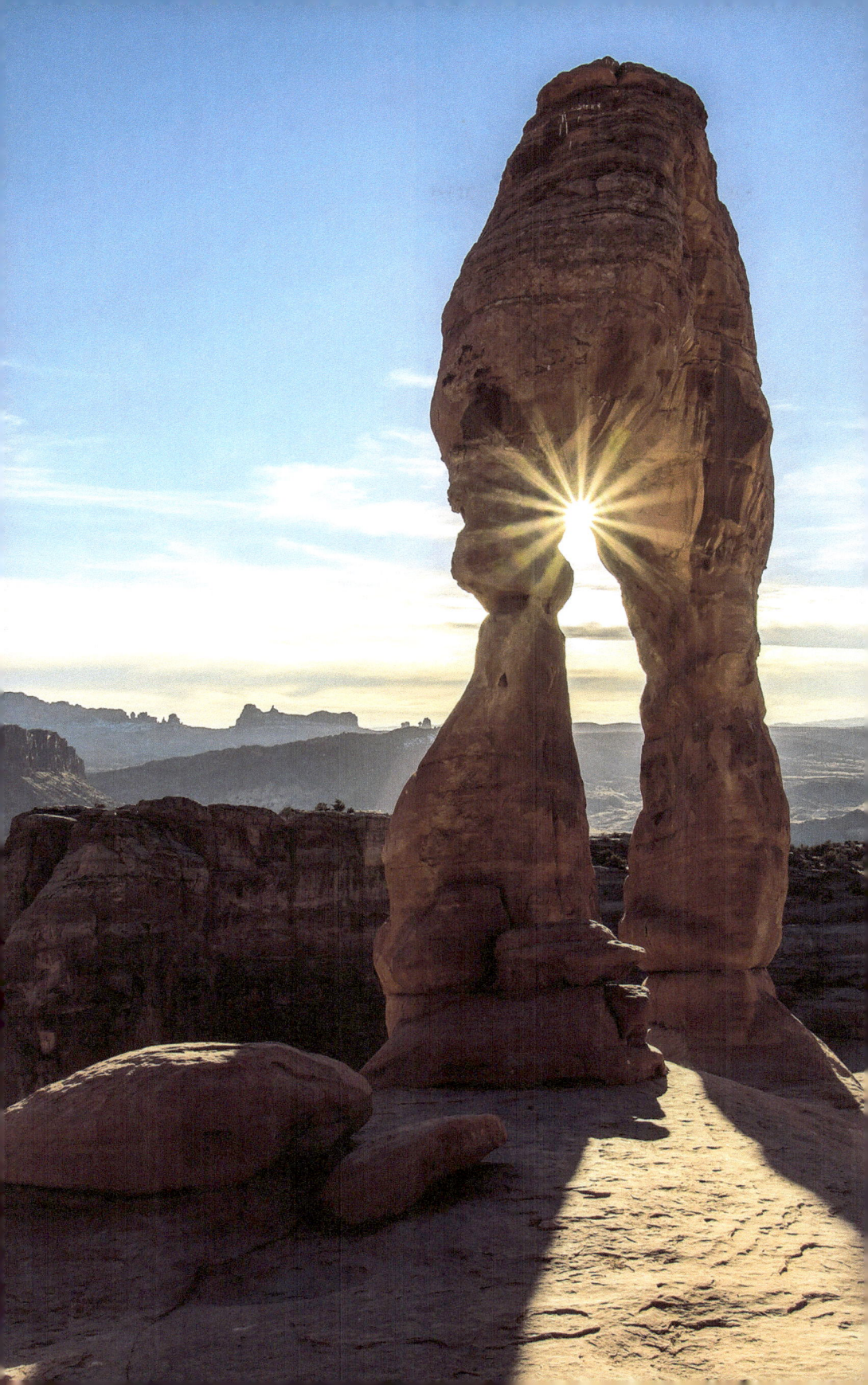

I can do all things

through Christ who

strengthens me.

*P*hilippians 4:13

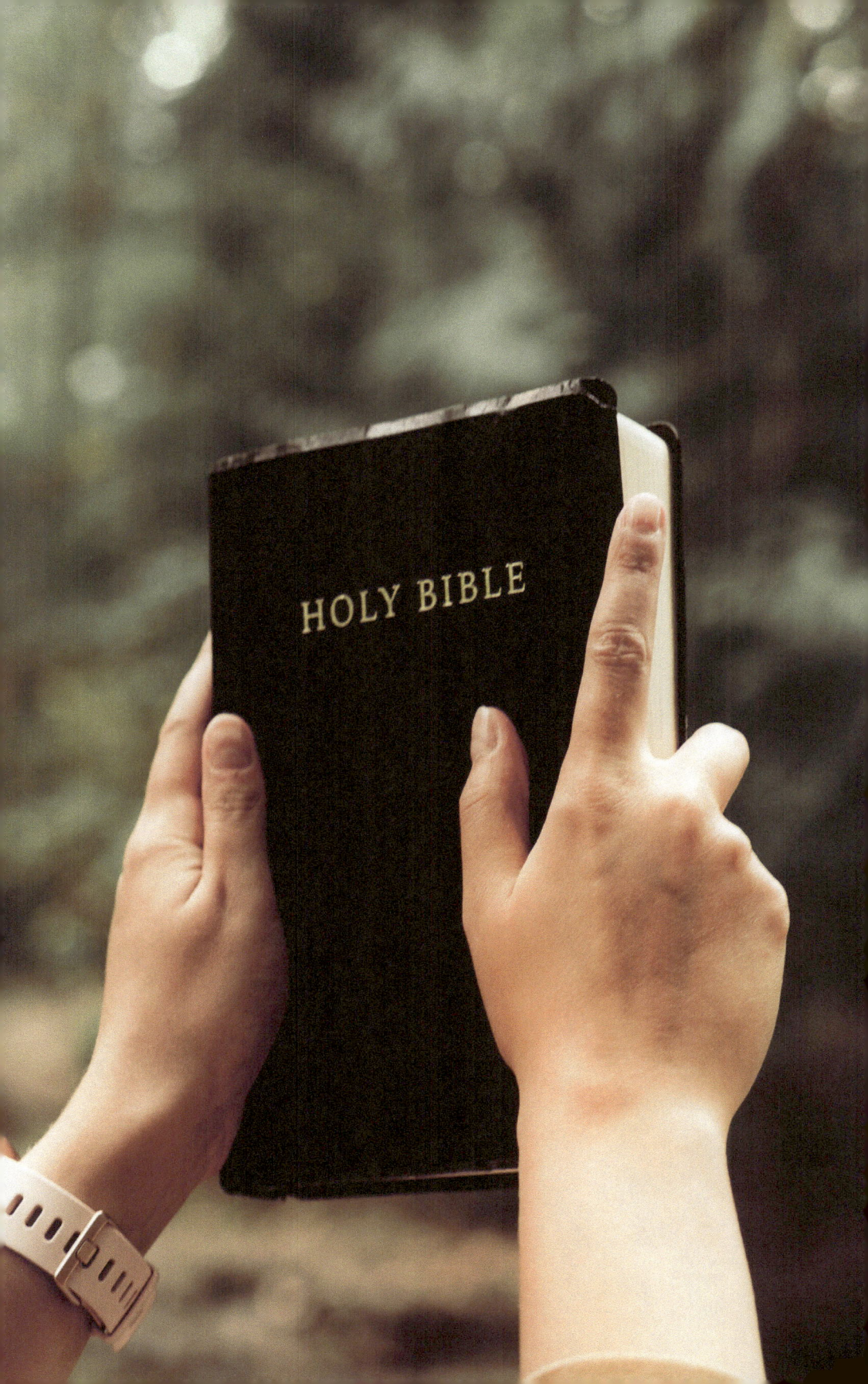

Fear not, for the

Lord is with you.

Isaiah 41:10

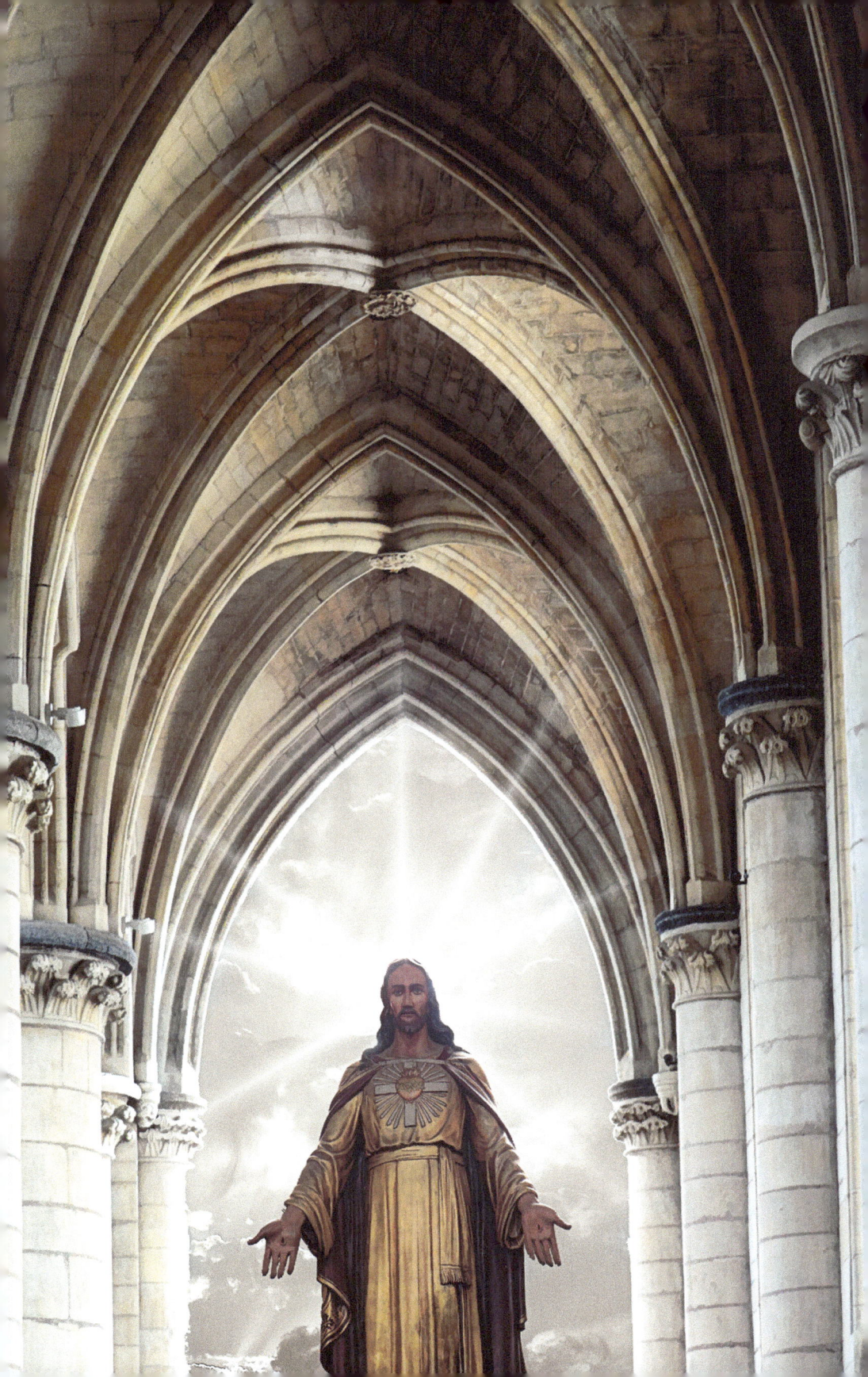

In Him was life, and

that life was the light

of all mankind.

John 1:4

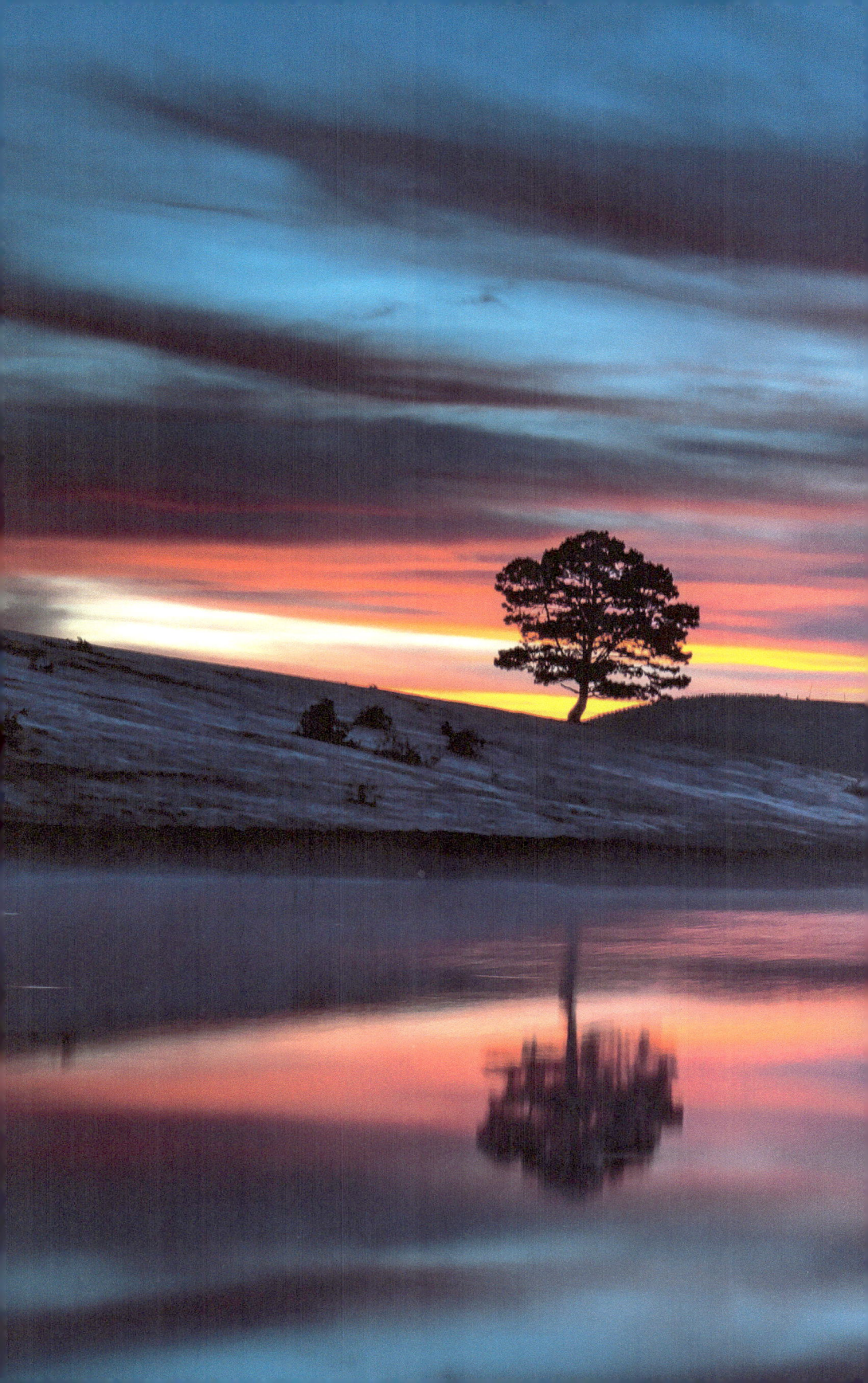

*A*sk and it will

be given to you.

*M*atthew 7:7

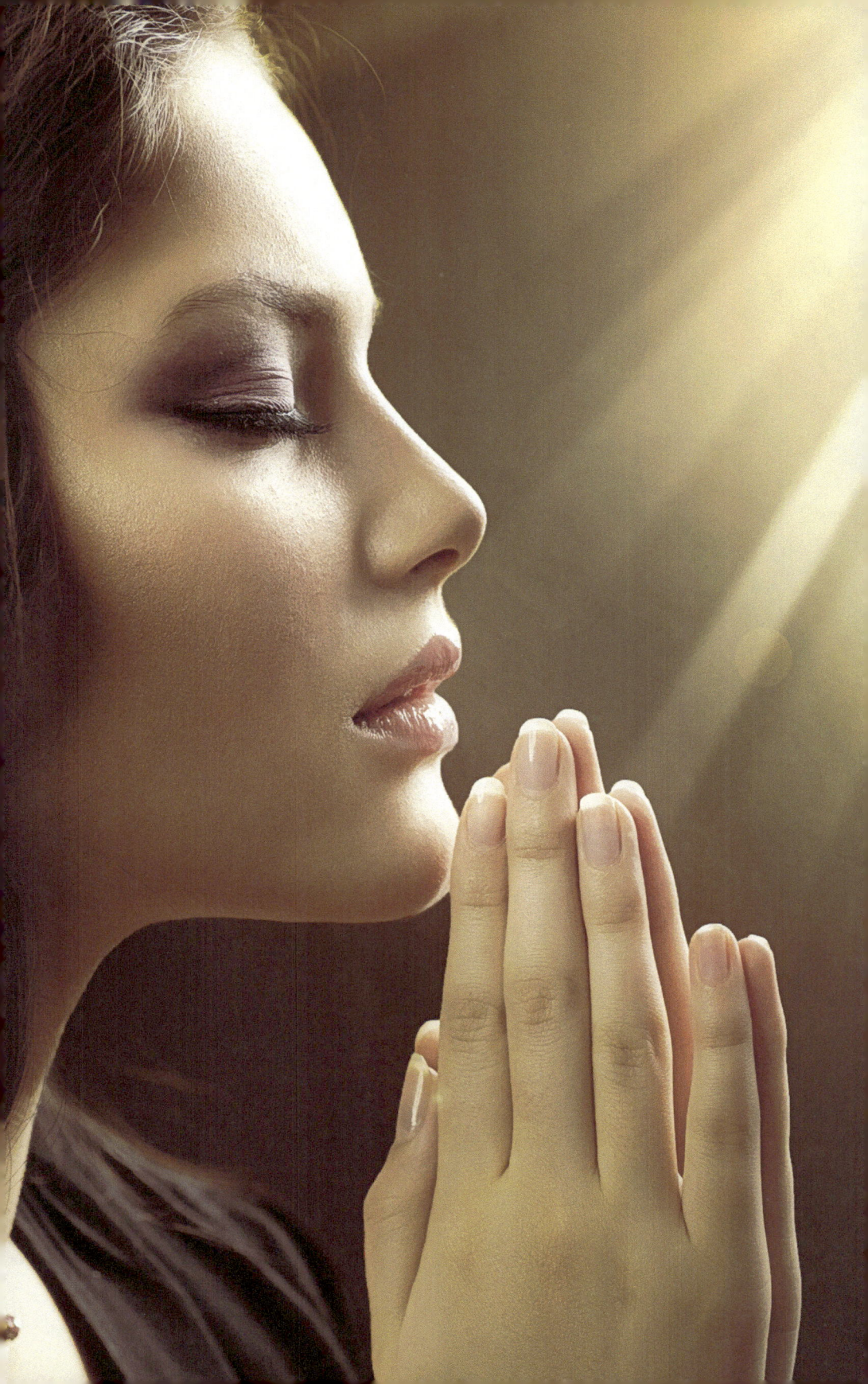

This is the day the Lord has made; let us rejoice and be glad in it.

Psalm 118:24

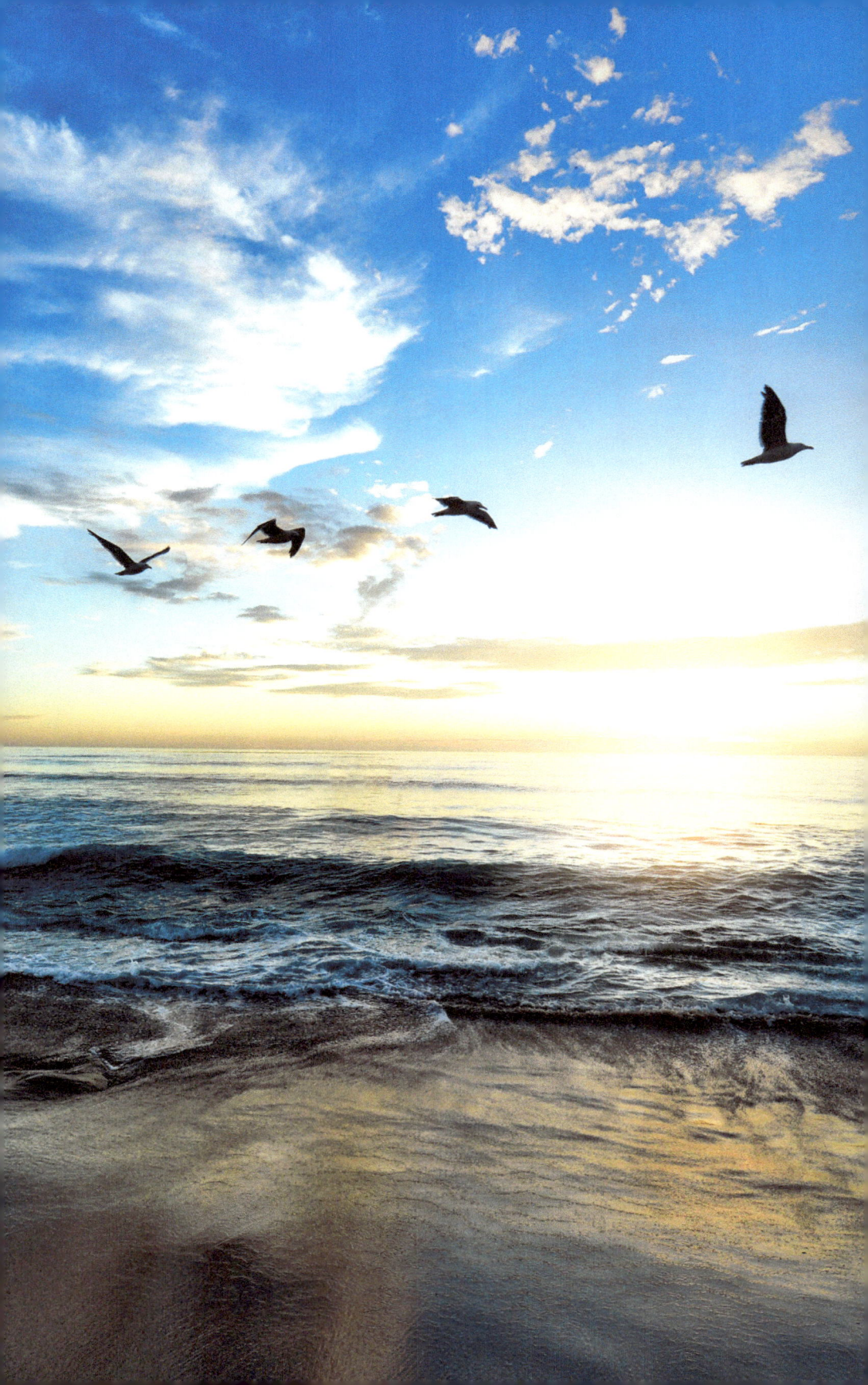

Jesus Christ is the
same yesterday, today,
and forever.

Philippians 4:13

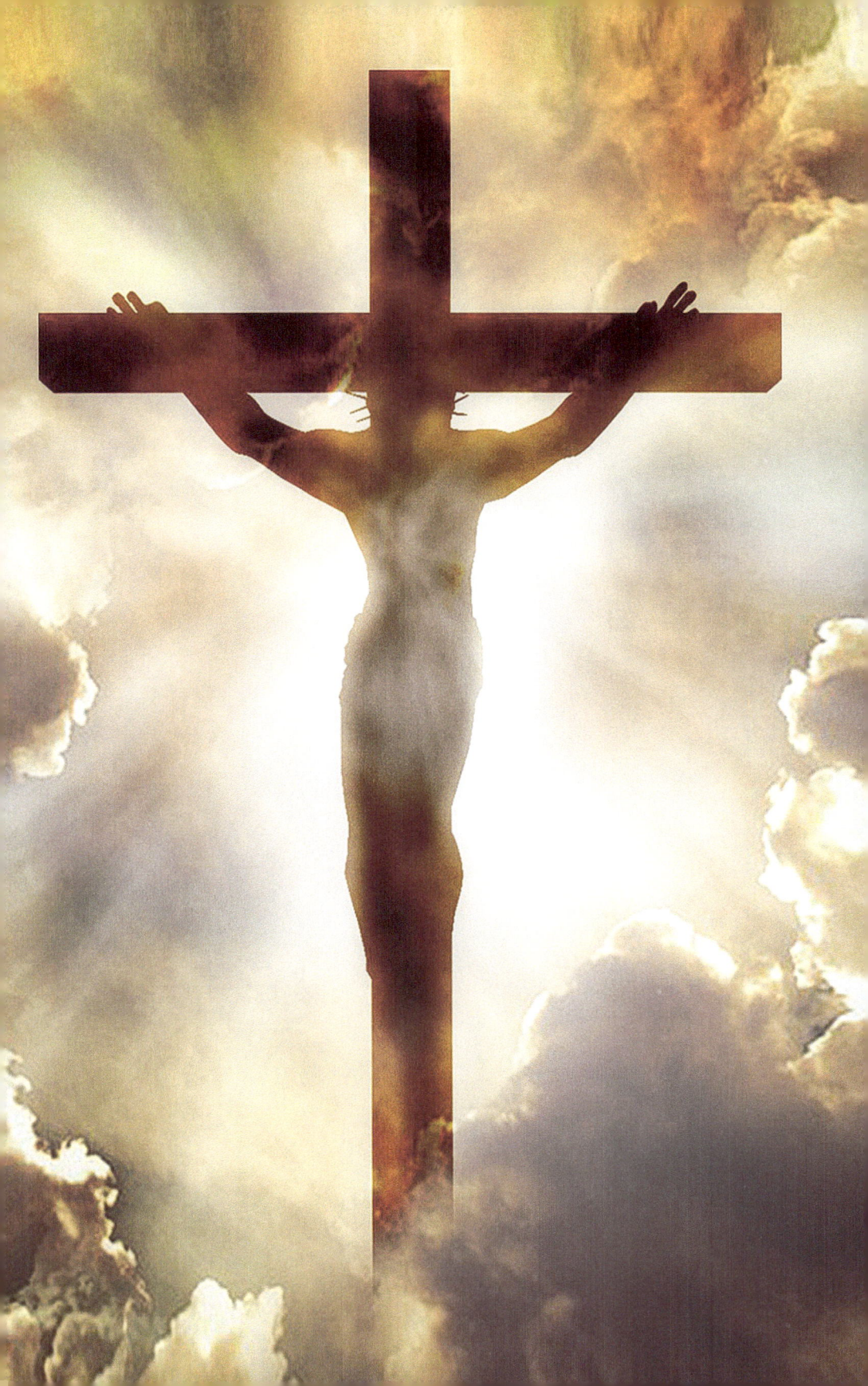

www.ingramcontent.com/pod-product-compliance
Lightning Source LLC
Chambersburg PA
CBHW050756290526
45792CB00008B/2214